# WHY DIETS DON'T WORK!

## Why you cannot keep off the weight permanently!

## Discover Freedom From Dieting Forever!

By:

Cody Horton, Ph.D.  Clinical Hypnotherapist
and
Daniel E Vance B.S. Nutritional Wellness, Physical Fitness

# Legal Notice:

**IMPORTANT: This book is intended to provide information and ideas pertaining to weight loss. It is NOT a substitute for professional advice from a dietician, nutritionist or your family practitioner. You should consult your physician before undertaking any sort of diet or extended physical exertion.**

**The publisher and author of this book will not be held responsible for any personal loss, health problem, or hardship that may come as a result of reading this book. We have made every effort to ensure the information in this book is accurate and up to date.**

While all attempts have been made to verify the information provided in this publication, neither the Author nor the Publisher assumes any responsibility for errors, omissions, or contrary interpretation of the subject matter herein.

**This publication is not intended for use as a source of medical advice. The Publisher wants to stress that the information contained herein may be subject to varying state and/or local laws or regulations. All users are advised to retain competent counsel and/or medical advice to determine what state and/or local laws or regulations may apply to the user's particular business or personal use.**

The Purchaser or Reader of this publication assumes responsibility for the use of these materials and information. Adherence to all applicable laws and regulations, federal, state, and local, governing professional licensing, business practices, advertising, and all other aspects of doing business in the United States or any other jurisdiction is the sole responsibility of the Purchaser or Reader.

The Author and Publisher assume no responsibility or liability whatsoever on the behalf of any Purchaser or Reader of these materials. Any perceived slights of specific people or organizations are unintentional.

This book and its contents (including but not limited to Entire Text, Artwork, Graphics, Photographs, Illustrations, Animations, Design and English Translation) are protected by the Copyright Laws of the United States of America.

Pursuant to Title 17, United States Code, this publication and all its contents is protected under the Copyright Laws of the United States of America. A copyrighted work may not be copied, reproduced, distributed or publicly displayed without the consent of the author or copyright owner. Any unauthorized use of this publication or any of its contents, in whole or in part, shall be considered copyright infringement. It is illegal for anyone to violate any of the rights provided by the copyright laws to the owner of this book.

Should you infringe this copyright, you may be liable to the owner for relief such as injunction, impounding and disposition of infringing articles, attorney's fees, actual damages and any profits resulting from the infringement, or statutory damages up to **$150,000** if the infringement was committed willfully.

For information regarding the authorized use of any of the contents of this book, contact the book owner direct. www.HypnotizeMyselfThin.com

# Contents

Cody Horton Ph.D.

# INTRODUCTION

## *Let us introduce ourselves first.*

### Cody Horton, Ph.D.  Clinical Hypnotherapist

C ody Horton, Ph.D.  specializes in cognitive-behavioral , Subconscious-Dynamic Therapy, Therapeutic Imagery and Life Coaching for creative and successful solutions tailored to her clients' specific goals resulting in dramatic transformation for personal and spiritual growth, career aspirations or breaking through personal and corporate obstacles. She combines a rich personal and professional background with her knowledge and practice of Hypnotherapy and Neuro-Linguistic Programming to address anxiety, pain management, sleep and eating disorders as well as habit reversal and behavioral transformation.

### Daniel E. Vance B.S. Physical Fitness, Nutritional Wellness. NFPT Certified: CPT, CSNS, ETS, WRTS

D aniel E Vance, author, nutritionist and weight loss coach who cuts through all the misconceptions about diet and fitness to help you transform your body, your health and discover your life again.

# Why We Wrote This Book?

Dan and I met through a mutual friend and in the course of events started a conversation about our passion for everything involved with weight loss, physical fitness and the attainment of both through natural and healthy methods.  After many late night discussions regarding weight loss reality shows we discovered our mutual interest in communicating our findings and our proven permanent solutions, and we hit upon the idea of writing a book that would put together our best ideas and attempt to shed some light on the growing national problem of weight management.

While, we certainly don't think that we are the only ones that have discovered the issue, we do believe that we can contribute to the national discussion regarding weight management.  Part of what spurred us into action is the plethora of weight loss reality television shows based on quick weight loss and seemingly easy solutions that happen overnight.

In a one-hour show, you can see someone lose hundreds of pounds.  There is NBC's "The Biggest Loser", LifeTimes "DietTribe", Food Network's "Weighing In", VH1's "Celebrity Fit Club", MTV's "I Used to be Fat", Oxygen's "Dance Your Ass Off" and, most recently, A&E's "Heavy". Britain, Australia and Canada all have their favorites too. "Celebrity Overhaul", Honey, We're Killing The Kids", and X-Weighted all covering the war on fat!

Some critics argue that some of these weight loss reality shows may encourage unhealthy practices in the name of rapid weight loss, inspired by the big prize money. Suggestions have been made about what happens off-camera, unseen by viewers, such as vomiting & purging by the participants. Remember, big money is at risk & your failures can be viewed by a national TV audience. YOU CAN'T FAIL!

There is also criticism that the large short-term weight loss will inevitably result in participants metabolisms being slowed down, leading to an uncontrollable rapid weight gain in the coming years. Of course we'll never see this long-term effect on our screens.

Another criticism of certain such weight loss reality shows is that they're far from "reality", in fact, quite deceptive. The role models provided cannot be emulated by viewers. The highly artificial environment of isolation, twenty-four hour supervision of doctors, nutritionists, fitness instructors & other professionals, many hours of hard physical exercise each day, removing yourself from the daily responsibilities of families, workplaces and truthfully..REALITY just cannot be copied by the general public. The reality is that the results of the participants' weight loss, on these television shows, can be reasonably argued that it is very short term, artificial and unhealthy at best.

It diminishes the true physical effort and psychological transformation that these people put forward to accomplish this and at the same time leads everyone to believe that all you need is a television camera with a national viewing audience and the weight just falls off....three months and poof, you're thin.

Our approach is for long term permanent transformation.  We both believe that everybody deserves the "Freedom From Dieting Forever."  We hope this narrative will help you discover a better way and find the permanent long term solution to your weight management obstacles.

You can find our individual weight and fitness information and solutions available at the following locations:
www.HypnotizeMyselfThin.com
www.FreedomFromDietingForever.com
and www.Facebook.com/HypnotizeMyselfThin

# CHAPTER ONE

# Why Diets Don't Work!

## *Welcome to the New Year and here you go again!*

E ven though you have not tried this program before, you are certainly no stranger to the yo-yo dieting that's been ruling your life up to this point.

Since you're here, there's a 98 percent probability that you're looking for another way to lose weight, this statistic is especially true for women, sorry girls. The boys however are only, around 60 percent unfortunate but true. This means that between 60 percent and 98 percent of Americans will be on another weight loss plan at one time or another during the New Year.

Dieting is an annual part of most New Year's Resolution checklists and weight loss is a high priority. This means that you'll set your goals with the full intention to drop every single pound, so you can strut around on the beach in a bikini, but then after the first week there you are, staring down into the bowl of cabbage soup wondering what the heck? What was it all for in the first place? Darn those New Year resolutions! So there you are, you once again failed the weight loss resolution part of your goal, but that is ok because you just write down another goal for next year.

**Rinse and repeat, and the cycles keep continuing.**

This sobering high rate of dieters shows us that we are all well aware that we need to lose the weight, but somehow every year we keep getting fatter than the year before.

Most people do not realize that diets actually make you gain weight in the long term, and that's become increasingly evident in the obesity epidemic that plagues our fast food, minimal exercising generation.

We now know that obesity is a national health crisis. Assuming current trends continue; obesity will soon outweigh smoking as the biggest factor in decreased quality of life, the added health care costs, and most importantly early death. One third of Americans are overweight, according to the Centers for Disease

Control and Prevention, and another third are obese, and getting fatter every year.

Obesity is accountable for more than 160,000 early deaths a year, according to a study in the Journal of American Medical Association. Society pays out more than $7000 a year in added medical treatment and lost productivity to care for the average obese person, according to researchers from George Washington University. For a person seventy pounds or more overweight, lifetime added medical costs alone can amount to as much as $30,000, depending on race and gender.

The urgency of this question: Why is it that the weight is so hard to work off and even harder to keep it off? Weight loss should not be so hard, but the cold facts are that it is. The simple basic formula for weight loss is well known: Eat fewer calories than you burn. However, if it were really that simple, obesity would not be the nation's main healthy lifestyle concern. Humans have evolved from an environment where famine was a constant concern to the current environment of convenience of ready fast food, empty calories, and lack of exercise. It is no wonder that, losing weight and keeping it off in the modern world is actually an extremely difficult task. This makes long term success in dieting a recipe for failure.  An alarming  review conducted in 2007 by the American Psychological Association shows that of thirty-one diet studies, it was determined that at the end of a two year period, as many as two-thirds of those dieters, ended up weighing more than they did before they started their diet.

We write this because we are tired of all the new fad diets that appear every year; you know the ones that are not to helping you keep weight off forever!  The ones that promise a healthy permanent lifestyle change.

The unlimited variety of diet pills available on the market are not the quick fix but a risky solution, as all have negative side effects. Do you really believe there would be an obesity epidemic if there was really a magic pill to effectively lose weight and keep it off? Astronomical amounts of money is being spent each year on these useless pills and fad diets, and consequently more of these products appear every year, but ironically people are gaining more weight than ever. Even though it is proven that they do not work.  It just means that people will keep on searching for that "quick fix", while these companies launch even more products for us to spend our hard earned money on!

Everywhere you look there are diets that are advertised online. As you notice they all have the same features in common: they all claim, lose 10 pounds in 10 days, lose 14 pounds in 3 weeks, and the promises go on and on. These advertisements play on your desire for quick results and support unhealthy or unsafe habits. The primary focus of these fad diets is to eat very few calories, which will allow you to drop weight fast thus making you believe their diet was successful! However the weight loss is just temporary.

## No "Quick Fix" yet after 150 years of Dieting

When you hear low-carb diet you immediately think of Dr. Atkins, however almost 150 years ago there was a man named William Banting who really invented the low-carb diet. Even years ago, people were saying hold the potatoes, please. They ate more fish, mutton, and fowl than pork for their three balanced meals.

We have been living with a 150 year obsession with weight and weight loss. Their term for being over-weight then was "corpulent" and obesity had not become the epidemic it is today. Looking back through history shows there has always been the quest for the easy fix for weight loss.

*Clemson University sociologist Dr. Ellen Granberg says
"We grossly, grossly underestimate the difficulty of
changing behaviors that fuel obesity. It is important to
show we're not dealing with some brand new, scary
phenomenon we've never dealt with before."*

History shows that William Banting's account of weight
loss, where he lost almost 50 pounds in a year, was by
knocking out bread, butter, milk, sugars, beer and
potatoes.  These were known as the staples of the
typical home.  He instead started eating more meats.
Thus his fifty pound weight loss. Banting's pamphlet,
"Letter on Corpulence, Addressed to the Public," was
introduced to America and became so popular, that
"banting" became the new word for dieting.

In the past few decades, we as Americans have
"ballooned" into an obese nation where dieting is an
everyday fight.  Our ancestors believed a certain
amount of plumpness would help withstand infectious
diseases.  It was also considered a prosperity status to
have an extra few pounds because prosperity also
meant more access to more food.  The amount of
exercise has been steadily decreasing over the years
with the introduction of mass transportation and cars.
It is much easier to jump in the car and drive a block to
the store than to walk and burn those extra calories.

The Philadelphia Cookbook announced "An excess of flesh is to be looked upon as one of the most objectionable forms of disease." With this announcement the diet fad craze had begun. Out came the expensive obesity soaps, reduction salts, and jiggler's to vibrate the flab away. There was even the laxative plan. The progression has only introduced even more miracle "fixes" for weight loss.

In the late 1800's the government put in their two cents worth and suggested to balance proteins, carbohydrates and fat. Years' later insurance company's claimed that being overweight raised your risk of death. Then in the early 1900's the Department of Agriculture built the food pyramid with our famous five food groups. Next began the charts showing ideal height weight ratios, which are closely related to the body mass index we use now. Diet foods and weight loss support groups soon followed.

Even with the weight loss history it is amazing that two thirds of Americans need to shed at least a few pounds if not more. This trend has even trickled down to our children. Childhood obesity has tripled in the past thirty years. New trends are showing that diet pills are being pulled for lethal side effects and weight loss surgery is on the rise. That being said, professionals are questioning if society and cultures are the cause of overeating and obesity. Everything is supersized from your candy bars and drinks; to your happy meals. It is no wonder we are an obese nation because of the explosion of video games, which has led to a sedentary lifestyle.

### *So, just how many diets have you quit over the years?*

Nearly every one you started would be the answer you would hear from most people.  Do you think you would be reading this if you were able to stick with your diet and exercise plan?

You most likely have access to several diet plans. This may be a low calorie diet such as Weight Watchers, a low glycemic index diet as a Zone or South Beach, a low fat plan like the Ornish Diet or a plan your health professional has provided for you.

You do realize that if you just start a wholesome eating plan and add in regular exercise, you will  lose the unwanted weight and your level of health and well-being will take off - not to mention the satisfaction with your new look!

If you lost only 10 percent of your body weight, studies have shown, you could expect:

- ✓ Increased Energy Levels.
- ✓ Lower blood pressure, cholesterol and blood sugars.
- ✓ Fewer aches and pains, less stress on your joints and muscles.
- ✓ Improved mobility and breathing.
- ✓ Deeper, more restful sleep.
- ✓ Reduced risk of type 2 diabetes
- ✓ Reduced risk of coronary artery disease (plaque buildup in the heart)
- ✓ Prevention of angina, the chest pain caused by reduced blood flow to the heart muscle
- ✓ Reduced risk of sudden death from heart disease or stroke

Suddenly work becomes more manageable, leisure activities are more fun, physical activity is more enjoyable, and it is easier to have a positive mental outlook.

# CHAPTER TWO

## Weight Loss Opens The Door To A Higher Quality Of Life.

### *So, how did you get here?  What made you realize that something had to change?*

D id you have the A-HA moment and decide that you needed a slimmer healthier you?   Whatever the reason, I congratulate you for taking the first step. You recognize you have a problem and now are taking action to do something to change it.

The first step you need to realize is this, "How did I gain my excess weight in the first place?"  You must address this question first, so that you are aware of the cause and avoid a repeat performance.

Did you start eating more?  Or did you just start eating the wrong foods?  Eating empty calories with no nutritional value can cause a major weight gain.  Most overweight people do not usually "eat more" than their "skinny" friends, it is more likely about the kinds of foods they eat.

Did your exercise patterns change?  Are you sitting in front of the computer all day?  Do you manage to get in a walk on breaks?

Did you eat from boredom?   Or was it because of emotions or stress that you caused you to start eating unhealthy?
Seriously think about your relationship with food. These are the burning questions that must be addressed to help fix future weight loss failures.

## *Try our diet quiz.*

*Even the smartest people have been deceived by the medical professionals and by the media when it comes to losing weight.*

*I know that when I originally started my own weight loss journey, I would have missed a lot of these questions. It's not because I am not smart... it's because the information available is very misleading.  Everyone has their own opinions of dieting and weight loss quick fixes, each that will sabotage your ultimate successes of weight loss forever.*

*This quiz is an easy test of your own knowledge and will possibly teach you something about yourself you didn't know. Hopefully, you will retain a tidbit of information that will help you on your journey to a healthier lifestyle. Enjoy!*

1. *Calories are the most important aspect of weight loss. The fewer calories you eat, the more weight you lose.*

   *True*
   *False*

2. *Dietary fat makes you fat. You must cut your fat intake down in order to lose weight.*
   *True*
   *False*

3. *Your hormone levels are not important when it comes to weight loss, especially if you are over 35.*
   *True*
   *False*

4. *One good technique for losing weight, while still eating your favorite foods is the "once-per-week junk food day". This technique, advocated by books like "Body for Life" and many others, can*

*help you stay motivated without causing your body any harm.*
*True*
*False*

5. *The older you get the harder it is to lose weight and firm up your body.*
*True*
*False*

6. *Your body needs a lot of carbohydrates, such as brown rice, potatoes, and oatmeal, in order to maintain health and energy.*
*True*
*False*

7. *Men and women lose weight differently. They store fat in different places; therefore men and women should diet and exercise differently.*
*True*
*False*

8. *It is possible to lose two or more pounds of fat (weight) per week and still be healthy.*
*True*
*False*

9. *There is no such thing as a universally "healthy diet".*
   *True*
   *False*

10. *Your mind is as important to your weight loss goals as the food you consume and the exercise you do.*
    *True*
    *False*

## Quiz Results

1. *Calories are the most important aspect of weight loss. The fewer calories you eat, the more weight you lose.*
**Not Quite!**

This sounds true for the most part, but it is actually false. While it's true that you do have to cut calorie intake to lose weight, there are far more important things than just calories when it comes to weight loss. For example, if you train with weights and put on muscle, you may need more calories than you are currently eating to lose weight, not less!  Muscle requires more calories to maintain it and maintain the calories burned due to exercise.

Another example is "post-exercise thermogenic response." "This is an extravagant way of saying that when you exercise, your body can actually absorb significantly more calories than normal, and they are not stored as fat. The result is an increase in body heat, known as "thermogenesis" which uses a greater number of calories than you can normally burn off.

This is yet another example; "I only eat four hundred calories a day and never lose!" If all you had to do was to cut calories, then simply eating less would get the job done. But this approach fails due to the fact the body's ability to adapt. Cutting your calories too low, makes your body think it is starving. This is not the result you are looking for. By "starving" your body you also slow (or even stop) certain hormones from being produced, these regulate your metabolism when calories are too low. Testosterone, thyroid hormone and leptin are three main examples. Should one of these three important fat burning hormones decrease, your weight loss comes to a screeching halt.

These are just a few of the examples why "counting calories" is almost a waste of time. Your body is not a machine; it is however a very adaptive organism that requires more calories on some days and far less on other days. Learn how this "caloric cycling" is the absolute key to a lifetime of enjoyable weight management.

2. *Dietary fat makes you fat. You must cut your fat intake down in order to lose weight.* **Not Quite!**

The theory that dietary fat makes you fat, is a common misconception. This could not be more false.  In fact, your body needs fat to burn fat! Balance is the key: the right kinds of fat, the right of amount of fat, and when you burn fat. Fat is your fuel. Fat is actually a much longer burning fuel source than carbohydrates. Fat has been shown in numerous studies to improve blood lipid profiles (cholesterol, and triglycerides), help in weight loss (fish oil, coconut oil), and make you feel fuller so you eat less.   Fat makes food taste better; obviously if your food does not taste good you will never stick with your diet plan.  You need to simply establish a diet that you can stick with and enjoy.  Eating the "right" kinds of fat is essential to your weight loss goal.  Make your diet enjoyable and easy to follow and fat will be your friend.

3. *Your hormone levels are not important when it comes to weight loss, especially if you are over 35.* **Not Quite!**

Hormones are probably the most important aspect of weight loss, and one that most weight loss books barely talk about. Without your hormone system functioning properly, you can forget about losing weight.  If you have low thyroid function (especially T3, the active thyroid hormone) you could cut calories to nearly nothing and never lose weight. Should you eat too little you can decrease leptin, this is a powerful fat metabolizing hormone found in fat cells.  Leptin also tells your brain, "Hey, I am full!  You can stop eating now!" This is very important when trying to lose weight! Fortunately, there are many natural remedies to hormonal issues, however you should discuss with your doctor if HRT, or hormone therapy is a better solution.

Top athletes use MACA to acquire more stamina and energy in a natural and stable way.  There are several studies regarding whether or not MACA really works to increase both your thyroid and testosterone production. Dr. Qun Yi Zheng performed tests on MACA at the request of the Peruvian government to once more put the benefits of MACA in the spotlight.  He found that MACA did indeed increase the levels of testosterone to form in the body to help build lean body mass. He also noted that thyroid production became more balanced. This age-old dietary supplement had been used by the Incas during their conquests in South America to obtain more power and stamina.

However, the most powerful "supplement" for hormones is short duration exercise (at reasonable intensity) combined with a protein diet, low to moderate carbohydrates, and healthy fats. Leptin receptors can be "reset" to normal, for example, eat a bit less on one day and eat a bit more the next day. Your body will never think it is starving and this also helps to keep thyroid levels optimal. Finally exercise (done correctly) increases testosterone and normalizes estrogen levels in men and women, creating the firm, toned look we all want.

4. *One good technique for losing weight, while still eating your favorite foods is the "once-per-week junk food day". This technique, advocated by books like "Body for Life" and many others, can help you stay motivated without causing your body any harm.*
**Not Quite!**

I do not agree with a "cheat day" dietary approach. In fact this is the worst way to diet, and certainly the most dangerous if you've any history of high blood pressure or heart disease. There are several reasons this is not your best approach for reasonable, enjoyable long-term weight loss.

To ask anyone to diet strictly for six days a week automatically lays great stress on the dieter. Believe it or not, stress is the main diet-killer! YES! Stress! Stress increases cortisol production, leading to increased storage of belly fat in both men and women. Stress also contributes to diseases such as hypertension and heart disease. Also, the mental stress of having to be "perfect" six days a week is just more than most people want to process. It seems like an awful lot to ask when you already have stress in your job, plus your family responsibilities.

Metabolism decreasing is another reason this is a bad idea. Keeping the calories low for six days begins shutting the body's thyroid production, in this case T4, which converts to active T3. Low thyroid means slow or no weight loss. Plus, when your "cheat" days roll around, most people eat so much that they shock the body. Their hormone levels start restoring leptin and then radically shift in order to protect against the sudden intake of calories. This change can cause severe damage to both your diet and your body. Eating lots of food in one day causes a huge increase in "inflammatory markers", or blood markers associated with a stroke, heart attacks and blood clots.

When you consume a wealth of bad food in one day, you feel miserable! Most people cannot even attempt to head to the gym the next day. They are exhausted. Their bodies are working overtime as they try to digest the massive calories. You end up feeling worse than your favorite foods can taste!

5. *The older you get the harder it is to lose weight and firm up your body.* **Not Quite!**

There is NO SUCH THING AS TOO OLD when it comes to fat loss and re-shaping your body!

A study published in 2008 showed a "reversal" of age markers within the cell when people began to exercise. But what was truly remarkable was that there were people as old as 90 years! Several studies done on men and women in their 80s and 90s show increased muscle mass and decreased body fat once a diet and exercise program is started.

Now the hard part is changing your mindset; *maybe not*. With the help of your subconscious mind, you can make the necessary changes to become a healthy fit new you. When you see results, you will continue... and this is true of anyone at any age.

6. *Your body needs a lot of carbohydrates, such as brown rice, potatoes, and oatmeal, in order to maintain health and energy.* **Not Quite!**

A dangerous misconception is that "healthy starches" such as brown rice, potatoes, etc. are the carbohydrates that are better for you. These "healthy starches" are easily converted into sugar by the body which makes you fat.

We did not begin eating a high-starch diet until about 10,000 years ago... Until that point we consumed large amounts of dietary fat, lots of protein, and raw nuts and seeds. We ate fresh vegetables and fruits when the seasons allowed.

While potatoes, brown rice or oatmeal have nutritional value, eating starchy carbohydrates in moderation is the key here for most people. And for some people, starches consumed in high quantity may be fine. But research has found that most people really do feel much better on a limited-starch diet. Vegetables and fruits are fantastic!  They are whole foods and it takes energy to break them down for food.   There is has been a lot written about the health benefits of Acai,

Blueberries, Raspberries and Pomegranates, so check out these foods.  An "apple" a day has proven to be very beneficial for weight loss. But we simply do not need excess starch in our diets, no matter how "healthy" it may sound.

7. *Men and women lose weight differently.  Even though they store fat in different places, men and women are the same from a DNA perspective and their cells will respond the same to exercise and diet.* **Correct!**

Men and women actually do store fat in different places. Specifically we store "more" fat in targeted places. For example, women tend to store fat in the hips, and thighs. Men tend to form fat around the chest area and develop "love handles" around the waist.

Just because we store fat differently does NOT mean we need to diet or exercise differently! This myth was created by the fitness industry in order to entice women into gyms. Men and women are the same from a DNA perspective. Therefore your cells will respond the same to exercise and diet.

Everyone should cut down on *excessive* carbohydrates and calories in order to shed the fat.  You should exercise with resistance (weights or with bands) so that you build and tone your muscles. Believe it or not, women should train with resistance the same way! Yes, it's true: women will not bulk up out of proportion just by lifting weights. A muscle either grows or it shrinks. You want your muscles to grow so you burn more calories at rest and get the muscular shape you want. You must workout for short but intense periods of time using 6-12 repetitions per set. The fact is; fat burning exercise is the same for both male and females.

8. *It is possible to lose two or more pounds of weight per week and still be healthy.* **Correct!**

Absolutely! I recommend 1-2 pounds per week as a reasonable goal for the first 12-16 weeks. Some weeks you will lose more weight than others, but this is a good average to start with. Also, I recommend nutritional supplements used to speed up the process even further by optimizing the metabolism and giving the body natural, non-stimulant-based nutrients that are both healthy and vital to weight loss.

9. *There is no such thing as a universally "healthy diet".* **Correct!**

"There is no such thing as a universally healthy diet!" This is 100% true.

Some people may find they need to consume almost all vegetable-based foods to be healthy. Not a problem. While others may find that the higher

fat and very low carb option works the best for both their health and weight loss, again, no problem. Still others may find that they need a high-starch diet. Just don't believe that there is only one diet that will work all the time. There are many different diets due to the way our body differs person to person. We'll help you find the way that's right for you.

10. *Your mind is as important to your weight loss goals as the food you consume and the exercise you do.* **Absolutely!**

The power of the mind to alter the body is an amazing tool to incorporate in your weight loss plan. Pro athletes use the technique of visualization every day to hone in their skills to make them excel.

For example, researchers asked a group of basketball players to visualize free throws. They did not allow them to practice the actual shot, but just to think about it, vividly, in their minds every night. After 12 weeks in a split-group test, where one group actually practiced and the other group only mentally practiced, BOTH groups improved their free throw percentages.

A select group of employees were told that they would lose weight because of their workload which was a totally fabrication. These employees were than compared to the employees who were not told this. Because the select group of employees believed the lie, they lost a significant amount of weight, while NO WEIGHT LOSS was reported in the other group.

# CHAPTER THREE

## What Are Some Of The Reasons We Eat?
### *We are creatures of habit.*

- ### *Emotional Hunger:*

U nconsciously we have accumulated many bad habits over the years. Sometimes we are not aware of the things we do until we consciously take notice of them. Think about it, what was the thought that led you to reach for a cookie. What was the idea? Were you feeling sad, distressed, or angry? When you feel the urge to reach for the cookie jar take a second and think about how you are feeling? What is going on around you? What mood are you in? At this point you can disrupt your normal pattern and form a new one. Instead of catering to your craving, wait four minutes, and then re-examine your need for that cookie. After four minutes you most likely will have gotten busy with something else and forgotten all about the cookie. This is because you have disrupted your normal pattern of behavior and have consciously replaced it with a new habit.

Happiness can also be attributed to emotional eating as well. As a child you were rewarded for good behaviors and this reward system can travel with you as an adult. The occasional reward is fine but make sure it is occasionally. Remember you have other ways to reward yourself than with food. Reward yourself with a trip to the spa for a nice massage, facial, or new hairstyle. Have a healthy afternoon lunch with friends. Unhealthy food does not have to be your reward which fuels your weight issues. Remember replace your old bad habits with healthier new habits by changing your mindset.

- **Boredom Eating:**

Do you eat because you have nothing better to do? Why not take up a new sport? Call a friend and go for a walk? This will be much more fun than eating junk food and sabotaging your weight loss goals.

- **Incorrect Hunger**

Are you really hungry or is there something else bothering you? There should be a healthy appetite that drives us to eat. When our body requires energy it is because our energy stores are depleted, our appetite signals it is time for us to eat. It is a simple reflex. We get hungry, we eat. Unfortunately it seems that there are times that our hunger is more psychological hunger than physical hunger. And when the mind is hungry, we feed it the wrong types of foods.

If you have eaten a meal in the last two hours most likely it will be thirst that your body is sometimes interpreting as hunger. If you know you just had your last meal short time ago, try drinking a glass of water, wait thirty minutes. If you are still hungry after this then a light snack would be fine.

It's about replacing bad habits with good because that's what'll make weight loss a permanent success. It goes far deeper than losing weight for its own sake but rather to arm yourself with the tools to make sure you succeed this time.

You need a permanent solution since you're reprogramming your mind and your attitude towards food. Look at it this way, it took years to form these bad habits so it stands to reason it will take some time to break them and create new healthier habits in their place.

Nothing is clearer than when we eliminate all of our favorite foods at once. Our body goes into shock, trying to override our good intentions and sabotage our efforts. Other diets bite the dust simply because we weren't aware of how we've conditioned our bodies over the years.

Your body is an amazing piece of machinery and will do everything to keep you from starving at any cost. This means that if you drastically reduce your intake of foods your body will shut down your metabolism to force you to eat. When this happens, you binge and gain back all the lost pounds and maybe more, you fought so hard to lose. Don't hate your body for it; it's doing just what comes naturally.

So how do fix this? Introduce changes gradually. Don't shock your body or it will frustrate your best intentions to lose weight. Why not treat yourself to a delicious warm bath?

## *Overeating Rewards and Affects Your Brain Like Drug Abuse*

*Ralph DiLeone, Ph.D. (associate professor of neurobiology and psychiatry, Yale University), lets us in on some very interesting research:*

*"Overeating rewards and affects your brain like drug abuse. That is what the brain rationalizes; the researchers concluded after comparing studies of overeating with studies of drug abuse, "said DiLeone. They also found that, at least in animals, sweet or fatty foods can act much like a drug in the brain. And there is growing evidence that eating too much of these foods can lead to long-term changes in the brain circuits that control eating."*

*"The food-drug link comes from the fact that in both the animal and human brain, there are specific paths that make us feel good when we eat, and really good when we eat sweets and fatty foods that naturally come with lots of calories". DiLeone says.*

*He further states, "Drug addiction is really hijacking some of these roads that have evolved to promote food intake for survival reasons.  That doesn't necessarily mean food is addictive in the same manner as cocaine but there is growing evidence that eating a lot of certain foods early in life can alter your brain the way drugs do."*

### Food Can Change The Brain

*Teresa Reyes Ph.D.,, a research assistant professor in the Department of Pharmacology at the University of Pennsylvania* was part of a team that gave mice a high-fat diet from the time they were weaned until they reached twenty weeks.  The mice received significant amounts of fat and became obese.  When the researchers looked at the brain's pleasure centers – specifically, the areas that change in drug addiction they found:

*"What we found is that in animals that were obese, there were really dramatic changes in these areas of the brain that participate in telling us how rewarding food is. The changes made these areas less responsive to fatty foods, so an obese mouse would have to eat more fat than a typical mouse to get the same amount of pleasure. And some of the changes didn't go away, even when the mice returned to a normal diet." Reyes says.*

*"So it is similar to what happens in cases of chronic drug abuse. The reward circuitry changes in a similar*

*way and that promotes the seeking of that drug, or in our case, in seeking palatable food." she concluded*

## Can Food Be Addictive?

More evidence of the connection between food and medicine comes from a team that wanted to understand how hunger can trigger an animal's craving for drugs.

*"Hungry animals will take a lot of drugs," said Uri Shalev, a researcher at Concordia University in Montreal.*

## Protein Data Bank

Shalev and his colleagues studied rats that had been subjected to heroin by pushing a lever. *"When the researchers removed the heroin, most of the rats stopped pressing the lever. But when the scientists also took away the food lever, the rats would press the lever hundreds of times, although they no longer received the food," says Shalev.*

The team began to think that the rats' behavior may have involved a chemical in the brain known as Neuropeptide Y, which makes animals feel hungry. And sure enough, when the hungry rats were given a drug that blocked Neuropeptide Y, they stopped pressing the lever.

Research at Concordia University in Montreal is now using the chemical to study the relationship between food and drugs in the brain.  Many other studies have also shown links between food and medicine.

A team at the University of California, Santa Barbara found that male rats chose sugar over small amounts of cocaine, while female rats did just the opposite. DiLeone However, the Yale researcher, says it's still unclear how far the food-drug comparison holds up, especially in humans.

*"There's an ongoing argument in my field whether food is addictive or not," he says. "But whether it's addictive or not, there are probably components that are similar to addiction."*

*"That means it makes sense to focus on eating behavior early in life, when the brain is adapting to a particular environment. It also probably makes sense to take approaches used to treat addiction and adapt them to overeating," DiLeone says.*

*DiLeone further states, "If you have ever wondered why it's difficult to stay on a diet, this observation is important to consider. The motivation to take cocaine in the case of a drug addict is probably engaging similar circuits that stimulate the motivation to eat in a hungry person."*

This new study of overeating and dependence was presented at the 2010 Society for Neuroscience meeting in San Diego.

# CHAPTER FOUR

## The Diets That Lead Us To Failure

### *Understanding Yo-Yo Dieting*

A part from the fact that diet has the word die in it, I don't much care for the word. Diet gives the impression of a temporary solution and with something temporary it must come to an end. When we reach the end, the old habits and the weight gain starts to come back again.

If you're on a diet to lose weight, you probably want to lose the weight for an immediate goal – something short term. If on the other hand you want to lose weight on a more permanent basis this is what we refer to as a lifestyle change. Think long term and lasting change! That's what you want from a truly successful program, as opposed to just wanting to lose weight for the moment.

Because diet is for the short term, once we depart, we gain weight again as we fall back into our old habits. This leads to yo-yo dieting as we jump from one diet to the next in the hope that this will solve our weight problem.

Like a yo-yo going up and down, so does our weight with every diet we begin. Every diet has the same symptoms. We start out and see quick results, hit a plateau, binge then gain back all the weight plus more.

Why do we get all the weight back plus more? Our bodies have what we call a set point. Think of it as the body's natural thermostat. It regulates your weight. As you drop weight after starting your new diet especially in diets that restrict caloric intake, your body goes into shock. Say, your starting weight before starting the diet is about 170 pounds. You lose five pounds. Then you lose another three pounds. Suddenly your weight loss comes to a grinding halt. So you cut calories even more, hoping to keep your weight loss going but again, you lose zero pounds.

Now, because you've limited your calorie intake, your body goes into self preservation; survival mode. This is where the Yo-Yo syndrome at its finest, kicks in. It overrides your body by making you sluggish and listless.

Now, you've the metabolism of a tortoise and you barely have enough energy to lift your own arm, let alone enough energy to exercise your body.

Yes, your body has taken over and foiled your attempt to lose weight. You don't feel like exercising to lose those pounds because you simply do not have the energy!  And to top it off you have an increased appetite!  Now your body adds a few extra pounds on top of that to store away for the next starvation situation you decide to go on! Because you put your body through trauma, it literally made you store extra fat because it thought you were starving.  Now it will lower your thermostat to safeguard you against losing any more weight when you try yet another diet.

*Nancy Snyderman, M.D., Chief Medical Editor for NBC News says, "The human body is smarter than we are, and is always adapting its metabolism-the rate at which it burns calories. When a person on a diet eats less, your body thinks it's starving and drops the metabolic rate to save calories and save energy." In her new book, Diet Myths that make us Fat, Snyderman says, "If you stop dieting, your metabolism is up again. The main side effect from going off and on diets is stretched skin, which tends to further frustrate the dieter."*

*Robert Jeffery, Ph.D., Director of the University of Minnesota's Obesity Prevention Center, agrees. "A person's metabolism-the energy we need every day is a matter of muscle. All body tissue requires energy to keep going and muscle tissue requires more energy than fat tissue. The more muscle a person has, the higher your metabolism. If a person gets older, the body tends to lose more muscle mass and then your metabolic action decreases."*

So there you have it, you only hurt your chances of losing weight by provoking your body into a defensive mode! Now it will make sure you get the added weight, just in case it is faced with the same trauma again. This information has been so well documented and this is why the phrase yo-yo dieting has become a household word. Your weight goes up, your weight goes down, your weight goes up again and then some!

There is a way around yo-yo dieting and the secret isn't shocking your body into retaliation, but rather working in alignment with it. I will explain more about that later in this book.

## *Fad diets*

If any of the diets you've ever tried in the past suggested any of the following then they probably belonged to this special category, and it's a good chance that it was a fad diet.

1. Promises are plenty of weight to lose in one week with little effort

2. Disclaimers that don't mention or recommend medical consultation prior to a diet

3. Suggest you remove entire food groups from your diet such as carbohydrates, dairy products or vegetables

4. Limit you to a set eating plan without considering what your preferences are, in other words, the rigidity of the diet is setting yourself up to fail.

5. Failed to reinforce good health and lifestyle changes

6. Reduces your eating to less calories than your body can survive on

7. Is the plan using sound medical information

8. Is the dependence of certain additions to the diet, or products effective

9. Demands over the top - unrealistic demands

10. Lack of scientific evidence that it works and why it does

Sound familiar? Most diets you know of fall into these categories. They rely on doing something drastic just to differentiate themselves from other diets whether eliminating entire food groups, eating certain foods on certain days, eat only one color of food or eating only one type food for days at a time.

Fad diets all have the same thing in common. Their solution to weight loss is always only a temporary Band Aid. A quick-fix solution to a problem that has been years in the making, which simply doesn't work. The fat that is lost after the diet is stopped will usually be quickly gained back.

None of these diets are sustainable and you simply cannot survive on them! The thing that makes your weight loss attempt a failure is the difficulty of adhering to such a strict diet in the first place. You go off your diet because of the lack of variety and boring bland food that you don't really like. Yes, you may lose weight, but the million dollar question is; what kind of weight have you lost? Any fad diet is an extreme way to drop pounds quickly, but the results aren't permanent. You often lose more water and muscle than fat, so not only are you destined not to lose the fat you want but you're damaging your health in the process. Any diet that eliminates entire food groups isn't good for you plain and simple!

We have a wide variety of foods to eat for a reason and this is because our body needs nutrients and it is only those foods that can provide them. Eliminating certain foods, means that we can become vitamin and mineral deficient. To cut out one or more food groups is setting yourself up for disaster. If you really think about it, this makes complete sense! A balanced diet consists of eating whole nutrition foods!

### Let's take A Closer Look At Fad Diets

The Atkins Diet, The Cabbage Diet, The Beverly Hills Diet, The Zone Diet, The South Beach Diet and unfortunately much, much more.

- ### *The Atkins Diet*

This diet has been known to be effective in weight loss. Subjects who participated in the program usually see fast results within a week. Participants have been known to lose between three and five pounds right out of the gate by increasing the amount of meat in their daily diet.

- ### *Why meat?*

Well believe it or not meat is completely filling and acts as an appetite suppressant.  Because of this, you tend to eat less for starters. It also encourages the body to burn fat in the absence of sugar. Because you are limiting your carbohydrate intake, (which your body metabolizes as sugar) you burn fat.  But fat isn't the only thing you burn.  The Atkins diet doesn't actively promote exercise and it works on the assumption that you will lose weight without having to some exercise. Does this make sense?  Your body needs some type of activity.  Exercise builds muscle and muscle is what actually burns the fat you so desperately want to get off your body.  Muscle and muscle building is a key factor in stimulating your fat burning METABOLISM!

In reality wholesome breads, cereals, rice and pasta actually help to increase the volume and mass in your colon which helps clean the intestines. Therefore to restrict your diet to just protein can cause constipation and even bad breath. Some cancers have been linked to diets focusing only on protein. No one knows for certain what the long-term health effects of the Atkins diet will have on the body. Only time will tell. In a recent survey, over forty percent of participants failed within their first year of being on the Atkins program because the diet was too restrictive. Keep in mind that you want to create health, and stay healthy so don't sacrifice your overall health to lose weight. There are better ways to lose weight and keep your sanity!

On a more positive note, the participants lost a total average of sixteen pounds during their first six months, but at the end of the year, this loss dropped down to ten pounds average weight loss. Results for almost half of the participants weren't permanent because people don't like to be deprived of food! We like to eat; this is why fad diets sabotage long-term success. The majority of participants gain the weight back in a few months because they slip back into old habits. Yes, they get back to enjoying the food they loved before they started the diet. We are creatures of habit so we have to create a different mind-set. Our brain and body are designed to keep us alive, so it's not your fault. We are not designed to eliminate entire food groups or eat the same thing over and over again, ad nauseam! As I mentioned before, your body is hardwired for survival and it will stop at nothing to preserve your current weight at all costs. Yes, even if this includes derailing your current weight loss program.

- ### *Low carbohydrate diets - why they're bad for you*

Your body is the master of efficiency in converting carbohydrates into fuel, so that you can move on with the business of living. Therefore to severely limit carbohydrates is unhealthy because the body will burn fat along with muscle. Yes, it can give you temporary weight loss but at what cost? And because you are limiting your favorite foods, it makes it difficult to stick to this type of diet. Brown rice, whole wheat (if you are not gluten intolerant), whole grains, beans and vegetables provide nutrients and fiber. Also when the body converts these foods into sugar, it is released into the bloodstream slowly. It has been found that oatmeal lowers dangerous LDL (low density lipoprotein) cholesterol. Focusing only on meat and dairy can lead to gout, arthritis, inflammatory bowel disease, diabetes, and more. Yes, balance and moderation is the key to successfully utilizing carbohydrates in your nutrition plan.

- ### *Low Fat Diets*

Despite what you may think low-fat diets aren't all what they are cracked up to be. Every human being even if you are Kate Moss needs a certain amount of fat in the diet. You need this for your body to function efficiently. Fat insulates your body and gives organs separation from other related organs. Fat coats your nerve cells and protects their wear and tear. Fat is also involved in important biochemical reactions, so to have some fat in your diet is important even within the context of the weight loss.

Fat promotes normal functioning brain cells, regulates the hormones, and immune system operation. It helps hemoglobin oxygen transportation, proper cell wall function, transporting and absorbing cell nutrients, etc. Simply put, fat is important in our daily diet.
These special diets are very popular because the thought is that if you eat less fat you will weigh less. Makes sense doesn't it? After all, fat is very calorie dense.

Before you venture into a diet like this there are few things you must remember; not all fats are created equal. This is absolutely true, not all fats are bad; there are good fats and bad fats.

- ***Poor Fats***

There is a link between saturated fat and cardiovascular heart disease. Cholesterol levels increase in the body by eating foods that are high in saturated fat and trans fatty acids (also known as trans fat). These fats are usually found in diets that are high in animal fats, which is why the Atkins and low carb diets are usually not the best diet. Diets rich in saturated (animal) fats are linked to certain cancers.

If your diet is high in saturated fat, fat deposits on your artery walls, restricting blood flow to your heart and your body. Your heart has a tougher job of pumping blood to the heart which increases blood pressure. Your heart may also increase in size to force the blood through your arteries causing angina, a condition known as enlargement of the heart. The increase in blood pressure leads to kidney damage and damage to the small capillaries in the eyes causing decrease in vision and possible blindness if blood pressure isn't controlled.

Trans fatty acids are some of the worst kind of fat to have in large amounts in your diet. Fats and oils that have partial hydrogenation are more than likely the trans fatty acids. This type of fat lowers the amount of healthy cholesterol (HDL - high density lipoprotein), which throws your system out of balance by increasing the amount of bad cholesterol present.

- ### *Good Fats*

In their basic elemental form they're known as monounsaturated and polyunsaturated fats. They play several important roles in hormone production and help to support proper cell function.

Fat containing omega-3 fatty acids, has been known to reduce the risk of heart disease, diabetes, hypertension and stroke.  Including fish and fish oil as a permanent part of your diet will augment your health for the long term. Eliminating the saturated fats as much as possible and consuming a diet in healthy fat will give your body the balance it needs in your diet.

Even if you limit foods high in bad fat you will still have a wide variety of food to eat while avoiding the worst saturated fat. Just remember, don't remove all fats from your diet, not all fats are bad for you. We need a certain amount of good fat in our diet for our bodies to function at their peak.

Changing your mind-set is the key to a balanced eating program.  Rather than embarking on a strict eating plan, commit to a goal of eating healthy for life.  When you begin to choose foods that help supply your body with the right nutrition, it becomes more difficult to eat the foods that don't support your mind, and body. In fact if you have eaten good wholesome foods for even a week and go off and eat something that isn't good for you, many have reported feeling sluggish, or ill.

# CHAPTER FIVE

## Factors That Affect How We Lose Weight

*There are several reasons for our weight gain.*

W hen you eat you consume calories and a calorie is simply a measure of energy. If you take in more energy than your body needs, it will store it as fat to use at a later date in the event of a leaner time ahead. But the problem now is that those times are few and far between. We live in a developed world which means, there are very few times when food really is scarce, so if we overeat the body will continue to keep storing it away as fat.

Compared with one hundred short years ago, you would be hard pressed to find any of our ancestors who suffered from obesity because they worked hard to eat. They'd either have to grow and harvest their own food or go to great lengths to get it. There was a certain amount of effort that went into the day to day survival;

they burned more calories than our readily accessible society does, where everything is at our fingertips.

Even what was considered a luxury item such as flour, sugar and chocolate, has now become an everyday staple of the modern pantry. Yes, these foods are so readily available to us and rather than use them as a treat, we tend to eat them in place of whole foods and also to over indulge ourselves on a regular basis.

As a result of this way of life, we are now left to find a way to get rid of the fat we spent years to pack on. If only we would look at our lifestyles and realize the answer is staring back at us from our pantries and not at the bottom of a jar of diet pills or the next fad diet that blows our way.

Understanding how your body works, how it burns fat, how it converts calories into energy, how you gain weight all contribute to your own personal weight loss journey. Educate yourself about how your body functions and this will allow you to make better decisions for yourself.

## *Why We Gain Weight*

We all metabolize our food differently. Yes, it can be frustrating to see people eat like a horse and never gain a pound! These people have a very efficient metabolism (the body's natural furnace), which utilizes all the calories (fuel) regardless of how much they consume. These people are the hummingbirds of our society and their weight remains perfectly controlled. But like the majority of us mere mortals, many become discouraged when they experience the opposite because of what is referred to as a "slow" metabolism. It seems that everything that is eaten goes directly to the love handles without any effort at all!

## *Slow Metabolism*

The metabolism is sensitive to our activity level and to the proportion of lean muscle tissue we have compared to fat. Our muscle burns calories for energy, therefore, the more muscle we have the more fat we burn. The less muscle we have the less fat we burn and the body has no other option but to store the excess fat.

## *Everything has a destination; it's either stored or burned.*

If we live sedentary lives, and we're not physically active our metabolism reacts by slowing down. When our metabolic rate is slow, we lose the ability to properly burn calories, and we store unburned energy as fat. That's why we gain weight if we don't exercise regularly.

People who are more physically active have greater muscle mass which burns more calories and therefore more fat. Some people are genetically predisposed to a higher metabolism and will always be able to easily burn calories. I know, it doesn't seem fair, but just because you might not be genetically blessed with a fast fat burning metabolism doesn't mean you cannot have one.

## *A Little Known Fact:*

Do you know that one person can burn more calories than the other person, sitting side by side watching a movie?  Why?  The person who is burning more calories with absolutely no physical activity has greater muscle mass than the other.  It is so amazing what one person can do with just a little more muscle mass!

## *Despite All Appearances – Your Diet Has Created a Pitfall!*

Let's say you lost fourteen pounds in three week which was your targeted amount of weight to lose.  What you may not realize, is that a large proportion of your weight loss is from the depletion of muscle and water. In fact as much as sixty percent of your weight loss will not be fat! This can throw your body into shock and have your metabolism grind to a halt!

This is the result of millions of years of evolution! If the body hadn't evolved in this way, thousands of people would've died in times of famine back in the days when there were no supermarkets or food stores!
By going on a crash diet and severely cutting back on the number of calories you eat, your body assumes that there is a famine, or your food supply at the moment doesn't exist, Now your body's metabolism slows down to conserve energy.  Your body simply doesn't recognize the difference between starvation and a fad diet!  Now it will start using your muscle for energy because of the lack of fuel (food source).

Muscle is very metabolically active (as I have mentioned before) and in times of need, your metabolism will use energy from your muscles to protect you from starvation. This happens for two reasons; one, your body wants to save its fat stores for when food really is limited and two, burning muscle tissue allows your body to require less energy to survive during a famine period. This is why if you establish a realistic goal, exercise to build muscle and eat to fuel your body, you will be met with huge success!

People have survived for weeks with little or no food i.e., anorexics, who are capable of doing this. However, if you look at them, you will note they have no muscle tone because the body is trying to keep them alive with the small amount of nourishment they allow themselves.

## What does this mean for you?

If you lose 14 lbs on a three week crash diet, you will have lost approximately 7- 8 lbs (maybe more) of muscle. If you continue with severely limiting your calories you will lose even more muscle. This is why many people who are severely over-weight will complain that they hardly eat anything at all. And this is true! They may have been on crash diets which severely reduced their muscle mass and now their bodies' burn fewer calories per day. This is why when you go off a crash diet and begin to eat normally, you end up fatter than when you started.

The reason I don't use the term heavier rather than fatter is because you literally are fatter and this must be brought to your awareness. It is impossible to reduce FAT levels, unless you work to increase your metabolism by building muscle and fueling your body properly. This is why yo-yo dieting is such a vicious cycle! All those people who are fat are not lying, their bodies have become very inefficient in burning calories, despite the fact they are eating so much less!

# CHAPTER SIX

## What Is Metabolism?

### *Let's look at it in greater detail*

M etabolism is defined as the rate in which our body burns calories. Your basal metabolic rate is determined when you are at rest. This is your RPM starting line; your decibel hum. Your body burns about 60-75 percent of its energy at rest.

For those people who have a slow metabolism many times the suggestion of "running around the block," sounds more like torture than fun. Many would rather sit, watch television, play video games or take a nap. The idea of exercise is to walk slowly to the kitchen to pull the curtains aside to see outside. When people are typically overweight or even obese, they are unwilling to engage in any kind of activity which promotes the added fat storage and in turn promotes the common problem of high blood pressure which is associated in part with high cholesterol.

One out of five people have what is referred to as the "metabolic syndrome." This is a serious matter, since this disorder can lead to an increased risk of cardiovascular disease, renal disease and atherosclerosis.

If you have any one of these conditions, you're at risk of getting a second disease or more. Obesity is also associated with insulin resistance, which means the cells have difficulty in responding to insulin. Some of the terms associated with insulin resistance are "insulin resistance syndrome" or "syndrome X."

## *Things will keep your metabolism slow:*

- Fasting and going without food
- Severely limiting your calories, i.e. a crash diet
- Snacking on sugar-loaded foods
- Sitting around all day
- Malfunctioning thyroid gland

If you are overweight and have hypothyroidism, are you at risk for diabetes? Absolutely!

Something called "insulin resistance" is involved in developing the various aspects of the "metabolic syndrome." The hormone insulin is produced naturally in the body, and aids in the transfer of sugar to the cells, where it's converted to energy.

When there is resistance, the body manufacturers more insulin, on the theory that if it gives the body more of what it is resistance to, it will balance itself out. Sooner or later your body just gives up and insulin resistance has won again. Now, your blood sugar rises, which can lead to diabetes.

Your body can't continue working under the stress you have placed on its organs. Now you have even less energy because your body's cells cannot convert the fuel properly which is glucose. Your brain requires glucose to function properly and remain healthy and get this, it uses 25% of your body's energy glucose.

You are also at risk for hypertension, dislipidemia. This is when bad cholesterol is high, good cholesterol is low, and your triglycerides are high, which contributes to the risk of heart disease, kidney disease, and a sundry of other diseases.

## Why don't diets work for people with hypothyroidism?

Hypothyroidism is a condition in which the body lacks a sufficient thyroid hormone. Since the main purpose of the thyroid hormone is to "run the body's metabolism," it is understandable that people with this condition will have symptoms associated with a slow metabolism. The estimates vary, but approximately 10 million Americans have this common medical condition. In fact, it is estimated that as many as 10% of women may have some degree of thyroid hormone deficiency.

Hypothyroidism is more common than you would believe, and millions of people currently have it and don't know it. Many hypothyroid patients struggle with an inability to lose weight. At first, if you've gained weight before your thyroid problem is diagnosed, you were probably told you'd be able to lose it more easily or told you'd lose all of your extra weight, once you started on your thyroid hormone replacement.

So you take your thyroid hormone, but the weight doesn't come off.  Now, despite "normal" TSH levels, a low-calorie, low-fat diet and exercise, you find yourself still gaining, or not losing weight at all. You may also experience having a high cholesterol level. When you tell your doctor this, he says, "Your weight problem doesn't have anything to do with your thyroid! You are just eating too much!"

Many people have gone on a 500 calorie a day diet, walking 3 – 5 miles a day and report not losing an ounce!

There are three factors that are against people who have hypothyroidism regarding losing weight:

- Metabolic Set Point
- Insulin Resistance
- Changes in Brain Chemistry due to Stress

# CHAPTER SEVEN

# Reasons Diets Fail

## *Calorie Count Error*

The wrong calorie count could mean gaining an extra 10-20 lbs. of weight over a one year time frame, especially for those 50 and older.

A recent Tufts University study found that these figures may be way off.  What?  It was found that calorie counts in fast food restaurant cuisine were off by an average of 18% and packaged foods were off by an average of 8%.  The study revealed that calories for some foods, including diet foods, were UNDERREPORTED by 21%, 28% and even as much as 200%!

## Hidden Calories Add Up

Tufts nutrition professor Susan Roberts, Ph.D., the lead investigator for the study, says these "hidden calories" are a real problem for people over fifty, who watch their weight. "Eating 10% more calories than you think is enough to cause 10 or 20 lb weight gain in a year."

## You Can Not Count On The Calorie Count

In fact, Dr. Roberts got her idea for the study when she couldn't lose weight!

From an AARP Bulletin:

*Roberts lost weight on homemade food, but when she was on the dining-out track she says, "I completely stopped losing." Suspicious of the specified calorie count with the foods she ate, she decided to test them at Tufts' University Energy Metabolism Laboratory. She and her researchers found about 18% more calories than the stated value in the food served in 29 quick-serve and sit-down restaurants. Of the ten frozen meals bought from supermarkets, there was an average of 8% more calories present than the stated value. Some of the dishes in the restaurants had up to twice as many calories as reported - other foods had fewer calories than reported.*

**Get this!  Many of the foods were sold as diet entrée's!**

The researchers also found that Lean Cuisine Shrimp with Angel Hair Pasta, for example, had 28% more calories than was indicated on the package, while Weight Watchers' Herbal Lemon Chicken Piccata had 21 % more calories than stated. The biggest calorie Bonanza was Denny's Meal with Butter!  It had a whopping 200% more calories than indicated.  You can read more about this in Dr. Robert's weight-loss book, *The Instinct Diet*.

This is troubling news, considering that new health regulations coming out will require a wide selection of restaurants to add calorie counts to the foods they sell.

But before you get mad at these companies, consider this; a 21% margin of error is still acceptable to the government according to current nutrition labeling guidelines!

This means that a 200 calorie frozen diet entree could actually be 240 calories.  That can make a huge difference in your weight loss program and could even sabotage your attempts to lose weight altogether, especially if you are eating a diet entree several times a week!

# Top Five Mistakes Dieters Make

You ate and sipped your way from Thanksgiving to New Year. The food was delicious, the eggnog and champagne divine. But now, well, now your pants won't zip up! Holiday weight gain is hands down the most unwanted gift of all. Here's how to avoid the biggest dieting mistakes and to start your weight loss plan right.

## *Mistake No. 1: You Crash Diet*

A restrictive and rigid course diet that promises huge weight loss quickly sounds good. After all, who doesn't want to let go of every excess pound you have in a few short weeks? And sure, if you drastically cut your calorie intake, you'll lose weight.

But here's the catch: You cannot eat like that forever. And when you go back to eating like you normally do, you'll get back what you lost, and possibly a bonus of even more.

*"The fundamental problem these diets have is that you cannot overload your biological drive to eat with determination. That's why 98% of these diets fail!" says Dr. Mehmet Oz, America's favorite doctor. He is better known as Dr. Oz, the host of the Dr. Oz Show!*

Any diet that eliminates an entire food group or replacing meals with mysterious concoctions isn't good for long term weight loss. If you count your calories, don't rely too heavily on those calorie numbers on your favorite packaged food or restaurant website.

### *The Easy Solution:*

- Eat a variety of healthy "whole" foods, so you don't feel like you are depriving yourself.
- Track your calories and find a way to eat just 100 to 500 fewer calories each day.
- Keep a journal to record your calorie intake and understand how portions can affect your weight loss goals. Keeping a journal is not a lifetime endeavor but can be a tremendous educational tool for you.
- Every long-term weight study that has ever been done in which people kept the weight off for more than two years comes back to this same basic rule;

- o Reduce your calorie intact by a small amount. It may not seem like it but 500 calories is a small amount. This way your body cannot tell you are on a diet, so you don't slow your metabolism down and this allows you to lose weight naturally and easily.
- o With a 500 calorie reduction each week you could lose one pound of fat.

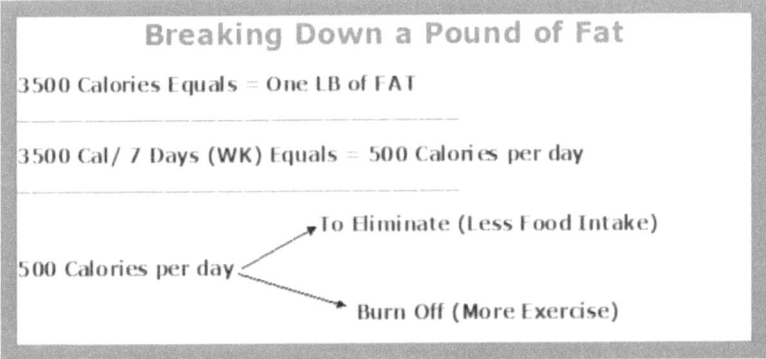

Breaking Down a Pound of Fat

3500 Calories Equals = One LB of FAT

3500 Cal/ 7 Days (WK) Equals = 500 Calories per day

500 Calories per day → To Eliminate (Less Food Intake)

→ Burn Off (More Exercise)

## *Mistake No. 2: You Skip Breakfast*

You think that circumventing your morning breakfast would be a quick and easy way to shave off some extra calories. Not so, because you are actually likely to consume these calories and more later on in the day. You may think you have extra calories to play with because you don't eat breakfast, so you supersize your lunch. You may also eat snacks that are not particularly good for you just because you are starving!  In addition, by skipping breakfast your body rushes to store fat instead of metabolizing it. In fact, research shows that breakfast skippers tend to be heavier. It was found that while breakfast eaters ate more calories, they also were slimmer, more active and had healthier diets overall.

In a study of people who had lost at least 30 lbs and kept it off, 78% said that they routinely ate breakfast. The reason for this is that they kept their set-point high, kept their metabolism working efficiently, and were less hungry at lunchtime so they ate proportionately better as a direct consequence of this one action.

### *The Easy Solution:*

Something to eat within 1 hour or so after waking increases your metabolism by as much as 10%. Invest in things like oatmeal sprinkled with nuts and raisins (Instant Quaker Oaks takes one minute and 15 seconds to make), a tablespoon of peanut butter, a vegetarian omelet with nine grain toast, or low-fat cottage cheese with fruit. A mixture of protein and fiber eliminates hunger through the morning so you're less likely to help yourself to the powdered donuts at the office or overeat later. In a recent University of Connecticut study, the volunteers had eggs for breakfast; they consumed 100-400 fewer calories at lunch than when they ate bagels, although both the bagel and egg breakfast contained the same amount of calories.

## No time to sit down to eat?

Try Dr. Oz Magical Breakfast Blaster when you travel to work or drop your children to school. *"It's fast, it's filling and has everything you need in the morning, say Dr. Oz. It's purple, so that kids like it too."*

*Magical Breakfast Blaster by Dr OZ*

*This recipe makes two 136-calorie servings.*

*½ large banana, broken into chunks*
*1/3 cup soy protein*
*½ tablespoon flaxseed oil*
*¼ cup frozen blueberries*
*½ tablespoon apple juice concentrate or honey*
*1 teaspoon psyllium seed husks*
*1 cup water or ice*
*Powdered vitamins (optional)*

*Put everything into the blender. Blend and drink.*

## *Mistake No. 3: Drinking Extra Calories*

Drinking extra calories is a national problem and if this is you, you are not alone. When you consume a large meal, your body tells you it's been fed and you fill full. But this isn't what happens when you drink high-calorie sodas, which are estimated to add about 235 extra (empty) calories a day to your diet.

How many sodas a day do you consume? If it is over two a day you are adding unwanted calories to your diet. Also, you body doesn't seem to register liquid calories the way it does with solid calories. Therefore after
consuming a jumbo-size soda, you don't eat less when it's time to eat again. Coffee drinks, fruit drinks, soft drinks, diet drinks, energy drinks, and alcohol are some of the biggest calorie traps. Alcohol is actually twice as bad because it overrides your willpower. When you consume a few cocktails, your willpower flies out the window and now that cheesecake looks irresistible. Later in this book we will discuss diet drinks more in depth, so please don't think they are the solution either!

## *The Easy Solution:*

Choose lower-calorie drinks. If it is coffee, omit the whipped cream, flavored syrup and drink it black or with a little sugar. "A teaspoon of sugar is only sixteen calories, says Dr. Oz. People aren't obese because of sixteen calories."

Can't give up your favorite soda?  If you want to drink your favorite soda or fruit juice, try using club soda as a base and then splash it your favorite juice.

## *Mistake No. 4: You Don't Snack*

Snacks get a bad rap because we think they are like junk food that we shouldn't eat. But nutritious snacks are actually a dieter's best friend; because when you eat more often it may actually help you consume fewer calories. Consider the fact that snacking keeps you from getting ravenous between meals and making poor food choices later on.  People who eat several small meals and snacks per day are more likely to control their hunger and lose weight. An ideal plan is one that uses snacks as half of your caloric intake. No one likes to be hungry so stop the threat of being hungry by keeping healthy snacks near you at all times.

According to an overweight obesity study done at Virginia Tech in Blacksburg, volunteers who drank a 16-

ounce bottle of water before each meal lost 44% more weight after 12 weeks than volunteers who didn't drink water before they ate.

When you feel a little tinge of hunger, drink some water and if that doesn't help cure your hunger then take a small handful of healthy snacks. Many times you may think you are hungry when in fact your body is really requiring water. A good variety of snacks are apples, oranges, strawberries, radishes, carrots and a small amount of nuts.

### The Easy Solution:

Every day, pack some healthy snacks in small containers or snack-size bags to keep in your car or at your desk. If you always have diet-friendly snacks on hand, you'll be less tempted to raid the vending machine or the refrigerator. Be aware of your portion sizes so you don't go over the top with it.

## Mistake No. 5: You don't drink enough water

Again, the next time you are hungry, take a big drink of water first, because you may not need to eat. Interestingly the hormones in our gut that tell us we're hungry are very similar to the hormones that let us know that we are thirsty. Our body is not very good at distinguishing hunger from thirst. This is why we usually reach for food when we really are thirsty. If we are not well hydrated, we can slow our metabolism down, which sabotages our efforts to lose weight by simply not consuming enough water. Water is crucial in burning calories. Adults who drink 8 plus glasses of water a day, burn more calories than those who drink less.

## *The Easy Solution:*

Drink water before each meal and snack in between meals. Often, hunger is just your body yelling for a little extra water. If 8 glasses of water a day seems daunting, try this mind trick; drink from larger bottles, so instead of fretting over trying to consume 8 glasses, you are sipping only 3 and half bottles all day long. There is no reason to always drink it pure either. Make the water more attractive by adding slices of fruit or a splash of lemon or lime to give it a different taste. We have clients that compromise and unsweetened ice tea.

## *Mistake No 6: Setting unrealistic goals*

## *Healthy Lifestyle Tips: Diet errors can affect Your success*

If you set unrealistic goals you will be setting yourself up for disappointment and failure. Men can usually lose 5 or more lbs. in the first few weeks because they have higher testosterone levels than women. Women on the other hand will tend to lose approximately 2 lbs a week. This is a good range to keep in mind. Keep your goals realistic because it can mean a defining moment and the difference between getting frustrated and discouraged or realizing success.

## *Mistake No. 7: Avoiding exercise or physical activity*

If you don't plan and engage in some activity, you place the entire burden of weight on your diet. If you are more active, you can eat more of the things you like - and still lose weight.

We have a client who was so uncomfortable and in pain from the weight he was carrying that he started out by just going to the steam room. He was committed to get into a routine and at the end of three months; he lost

30 pounds just by visiting the steam room and Jacuzzi. That enabled him to start on a regular exercise plan and has now lost another 30 pounds.  That is 60 pounds total!

# CHAPTER EIGHT

## One Word Makes Weight Loss Easier
### *Understanding The Positive Power Of "Do"*

O ne of the reasons people have such disastrous results with restrictive diets is that the diets all about what _not_ to eat.

A recent friend's experience on the tennis court made me think about this. Every day he struggles to improve his tennis game. Recently he began working with master tennis coach Jerry White, the head pro at LA Fitness Tennis Club.  Every time he misses a ball, hits a crummy serve, or screws up what should be a simple put-away, he tells his trainer all the things he thought he was doing wrong. "I don't follow through!"  "I hit the ball too late!"  "I didn't have my racket back in time!"  "My feet were in the wrong position."  And on and on.

His trainer replied: "Stop thinking about all the things you shouldn't do. Concentrate on the things to do correctly instead."

So instead of filling his already cluttered brain with "don'ts" he began to think about positive things, like hitting the ball in the middle of the racket, or throwing the ball higher.

## Which Reminds Me Of The Power Of NO!

We fill our minds with a lot of negative thoughts about food. "Don't eat carbs" "Don't eat saturated fat" "Stay away from trans-fat" "Don't eat late at night" "Don't eat this way" "Don't eat that way" "Don't" "Don't" "Don't!" We put so much of our mental energy in what _not_ to do instead of concentrating on the positive things we can do to control our diet and weight. What if we start from the premise of a list of "do's" instead of spending all that energy on a list of "don'ts"?

For example: Eat berries and nuts. Drink plenty of water. Eat protein. Doesn't it have a different psychic "feel" to it than "Don't eat bagels" The key is finding a positive re-enforcement you enjoy.

Concentrating on what is positive instead of what not to do may seem like a small difference, but it is actually huge. Your brain and the subconscious, works in mysterious ways. Brain scans of a person thinking of an orange look the same as brain scans of a person actually looking at an orange. This indicates that, at least on some level, the brain cannot distinguish between what's physically there and what's imagined. Your mind's imagination is as strong as reality, as any Olympian athlete can attest.

If you put your mental energy toward a negative action (like not eating food fast), you're actually giving the negative action mental currency and power! You are adding a lot of attention and focus on exactly what you're trying to ***stop*** doing. When you focus on an object, like a food, the brain isn't any good at figuring this out, it doesn't think, "Hey, he really means he doesn't want to eat this food." Rather, it reinforces you to think only about the food. Your mind doesn't understand the word don't, all it knows is what you are thinking about so you end up doing exactly what you are trying not to do. A positive reinforcement is just as strong and powerful as a negative thought so continue to be aware of what you are reinforcing.

Just like my friend the tennis player think about what you do want, not what you don't want. Personally, we find it much easier and ultimately more productive to think "I will eat some berries" than to put mental energy and focus on a thought like "I won't eat a pint of Cherry Garcia."

So why not fool your brain by thinking about the food you want included in your diet rather than those which you don't want to include?

# THAT IS THE POWER OF "DO!"

# CHAPTER NINE

## I Hate To Exercise!

### *I Don't Need No Stinking Exercise!*

This seems to be the crux of the matter, akin to the requirement of AA, that you submit to a higher power.  Of all the people in the world, those with a slow metabolism, need to exercise. It makes some people tired just thinking about exercise and they continue to resist the very thing that will set them on their course. Get in the Game!  Find an activity that you think would be fun and get moving because there is no way around it, you cannot lose weight and you cannot be healthy without exercising. Your body needs it! It clamors for it! And if you ignore its demands, it'll begin to reinforce those demands with joint pain and stiffness, heart disease, people guessing your age as 10-20 years older than you are; weakness; tiredness, mental fogginess and more. You know you should do, so make a contract with yourself that you want to engage in some activity every day. Like Nike's slogan says: *Just do it*. Don't think about it, *just do it*. This is where the power of the mind is a key to your success and we will address this in a little bit on how to accomplish this.

## In What Other Ways Can I Speed Up My Metabolism?

As you might guess, the way to speed up your metabolism is as described above along with eating sensible meals, getting some exercise, and getting adequate sleep will improve your life exponentially. It also helps in your ability to quickly go to sleep and staying asleep, until it's time to wake up.

Also, have your thyroid checked and if you are taking medication, consult your pharmacist or doctor about the side effects of what you are taking.

## Things to avoid:

Be aware of over-the-counter pills that promise to increase metabolism. Some are harmless, but others contain animal thyroid extract and can give you diarrhea, excessive sweating, trembling, increased heart rate, and protruding eyes.

**Skipping meals:** This is disastrous! Eat three good wholesome meals a day with snacks in between.

**Neglecting your water:** Fill one to three bottles with a small amount of water then freeze. The next day, fill the bottles up with cold water and carry them with you. If you choose flavored water sold in supermarkets, be sure to read the label before you buy it.

### *The Disastrous Effects Of Dieting . . . . .*

## Stop!!!   If you read nothing else please read this!  This is so important!

Your body will adapt to the low number of calories by changing the chemicals it produces to ensure that you stay alive during the famine (be it real or just a diet!). The body increases the amount of fat storage enzymes and decreases the amount of fat-burning enzymes. This also reduces the amount of thyroid hormones that regulate your metabolism.

The body adapts to survive on fewer calories by slowing down the number of calories you burn each day (aka metabolism). This means that you would come to a point where to lose more fat you will have to cut calories to a ridiculously low level.  Not only will it almost impossible to maintain but also muscle loss and decrease in metabolic rate would mean a rapid increase in weight is more likely. Even if you're the most hardened dieter you'll have to relapse back to higher calories and your body is very vulnerable to rapid weight gain, when this happens.

Low calorie diets are extremely difficult to maintain! Your body is literally screaming at you to go and find something to eat. What also happens, is that after a long time of not eating, that you skipped lunch or had no dinner in the evening is often the case when on a low calorie diet, you'll immediately gorge on the first thing you can find . This is often something unhealthy and usually something that's full of sugar and saturated fat.

Your body will immediately turn this into fat (and it'll often contain a lot of calories) as it hasn't had any energy for so long and it'll assume it'll not receive anything in a long time after the meal. Your body is really behaving like it has a mind of its own! This should be obvious now, but to keep the fat loss effective, starving yourself isn't an option.

**Exercise is important! Low calorie diets also makes so exercise is difficult because you simply do not have enough energy.**

# Metabolism & Enzymes

Metabolism is the chemical reaction that occurs in living organisms to sustain life. This is the process that organisms utilize to grow, reproduce, maintain their structures and respond to their environment. *Metabolism is usually divided into two categories:*

- Catabolism breaks organic material, for example to harvest energy in cellular respiration.
- Anabolism, however, uses energy to create components of cells such as proteins and nucleic acids.

The metabolism of an organism determines which substances it'll find useful and what it will find poisonous. The speed of metabolism affects the fat metabolism and governs how much food an organism will require.

## *The benefit of enzymes:*

- The chemical reactions of metabolism are organized into metabolic pathways, where a chemical is transformed into another by a sequence of enzymes.
- Enzymes are crucial to metabolism because they allow organisms to drive desirable but thermodynamically unfavorable reactions by coupling them to favorable ones, and because they act as catalysts to allow these reactions to proceed quickly and efficiently.
- Enzymes also allow the regulation of metabolic pathways in response to changes in the cell's environment or signals from other cells.

# CHAPTER TEN

# The Risk Of Getting Diabetes

*Do You Need Any More Motivation Than The Risk For Type 2-Diabetes?*

D iabetes is a disease in which blood glucose levels are higher than normal. People with diabetes have problems converting food to energy. After a meal, food is broken down into a sugar called glucose, which is transported by the blood to cells throughout the body. Cells use the hormone insulin, made in the pancreas, to help them process blood glucose into energy.

People develop type 2-diabetes because the cells in muscle, liver and fat don't use insulin properly. Eventually, the pancreas doesn't make enough insulin for the body's needs. As a result, the amount of glucose in the blood increases while the cells are starved of energy.

Over the years high blood sugar damages nerves and blood vessels, leading to complications such as heart disease, stroke, blindness, kidney disease, nerve problems, gum infections, impotence, nerve loss, dementia and amputation. Quite a list and it is life threatening in addition to being a national epidemic.

## *Can type 2-Diabetes be prevented?*

Research has shown that people at risk for type 2-diabetes can prevent or slow the development of type 2-diabetes by losing a little weight. The results of the Diabetes Prevention Program (DPP) show that weight loss through moderate diet changes and physical activity can delay and prevent type 2-diabetes.

This federally funded study of 3,234 people at high risk for diabetes who experienced a 5-7% weight loss was able to circumvent taking type 2-diabetes.  For example if a person weighing 200 lbs lost 10-14 lbs (5-7%) they would balance out their glucose levels.

Family history and obesity are strong risk factors for type 2-diabetes.
DPP studied participants who were overweight and had higher than normal levels of blood glucose.  DPP

referred to this condition as pre-diabetes or also, impaired glucose tolerance.

Both pre-diabetes and obesity are strong risk factors for type 2-diabetes. Because of the high risk of diabetes among some minority groups, about half of the DPP participants were African American, Alaska Native American Indian, Asian American, Pacific Islander, or Hispanic Latino.  Others DPP participants at high risk for developing type 2-diabetes, were women with a history of gestational diabetes and individuals aged 60 or older.

DPP tested three approaches to preventing diabetes:

- Lifestyle Change.
  - A program of healthy eating and physical activity.
  - People in the lifestyle change group who increased their activity approximately 30 minutes a day, 5 days a week (usually by walking), and began a healthy eating program showed a reduced risk of 71 percent.

- Diabetes Drug Metformin.
    - The second group who took the diabetes drug Metformin showed a reduced risk of 31 percent.

In the first year of study, the participants lost an average of fifteen pounds. Lifestyle change was even more effective in those aged sixty and older.

# Calculate Your Desired Calories

The first step is to keep your metabolism up. Be sure that your diet contains at least 10 calories per lb of your ideal weight. For example: if you want to weigh 150 lbs, then you should be eating at least 1500 calories. With this formula, your weight loss will happen gradually, but you will not slow down your metabolism and consequently you will be able to keep your set-point high.

*Ideal Weight x 10 Calories = Calorie Intake*
*120 X 10 Calories = 1200 Calories*
*150 X 10 Calories = 1500 Calories*
*180 X 10 Calories = 1800 Calories*

Of course there are more complicated approaches to calculating your caloric requirements for weight management. But the above equation is simplest.

### The BMR Formula

The **BMR formula** uses the variables of height, weight, age and gender to calculate the Basal Metabolic Rate (BMR). This is more accurate than calculating calorie need based on body weight alone. The only factor it omits is lean body mass (the ratio of muscle-to-fat). Remember, leaner bodies need more calories than less leaner ones. Therefore, this equation will be very accurate in all but the very muscular (which under-estimates calorie needs) and the very fat (which over-estimates calorie needs).

### Why Estimate Your Caloric Needs?

To estimate how many calories you should consume in order to *maintain your weight*, you'll need to do a little math. By using a simple formula called the Harris-Benedict principle, you can assess your Basal Metabolic rate also known as your BMR.

After you calculate your ideal calorie intake, you may need to cut calories or exercise to burn your fat stores.

Then you use this formula to maintain your ideal weight.

## BMR Calculations

http://www.bmi-calculator.net/bmr-calculator/

### The Harris Benedict Equation

http://www.bmi-calculator.net/bmr-calculator/harris-benedict-equation/

I trust now that your thoughts to drastically reduce your caloric intake are removed from your mindset and you are eager to learn the ideal way to a leaner, sexier and healthier new you!

It is our belief that this information is important from an educational standpoint. It will help you formulate a plan using the foods you enjoy while losing weight. But, as you progress and adopt a healthy lifestyle you won't focus on calorie counting as the end all to solve your weight loss problems. No, the solution lies in changing your lifestyle to enjoy what you eat.

# CHAPTER ELEVEN

# Diet Myths That Are Simply Not True

### *The Truth Can Set You Free*

### *Diet Myth #1*

> o   You can reduce belly fat by doing
>     crunches, and sit ups to reveal rock hard
>     abs. You often see these infomercials for
>     AB machines, claiming that by doing them
>     every day you will eliminate all the fat
>     around your middle region. No more
>     hanging gut! Now, if only it were that
>     simple!

The truth is that these don't work! You cannot lose fat from one area of the body alone; your body doesn't work like that. When you store the fat, it stores it all over the body!  By the same token when you lose fat, you lose it all over!  Again, you never lose fat in just one place alone!

If you do dumbbell curls every day for months on just one arm, what do you think would happen? You would end up with a very muscular arm and would probably look pretty lopsided.  There would still be the same amount of fat in both arms: This does vary from person to person, ***but it still doesn't negate the fact you cannot spot reduce.***

Now, I am not suggesting that it doesn't do any good to do crunches, or use ab machines, because it does build muscle, and as I mentioned before conditioned muscle burns calories.  However, if you think just by doing certain exercises you will burn the fat in that specific area, you will set yourself up for failure.  You will still have a layer of fat resting on top of that beautiful muscle.  The way to burn calories and fat is to eat properly, exercise properly to accelerate your metabolism for a healthy lifestyle change and not a quick fix.

So if you want those six pack abs to show you want to lose the fat.  Your stomach muscles are a small muscle group and yes, you can build them up fairly easily by training sometimes only once a week.  The key is to do an overall body workout to lose that stomach fat so you can show off those killer abs!

Keep in mind that if your body fat is too low, it can interfere with the body to function properly, i.e. women's menstrual cycle; ability to think properly; to have energy and so on.

## *Diet Myth #2*

- o The common myth that people think is that fat and muscle is interchangeable.

When I began lifting weights my friends all said, "When you stop lifting weights all the muscle you have in your body will morph into fat and you will look awful.

The truth is muscle ***cannot*** be converted into fat and fat cannot turn into muscle! So this fear is totally un-warranted. One of my friends revealed that they had not lifted weights because the fear was that this myth was true.

One of my friends who is a famous bodybuilder stopped training and lifting weights. Months later his body did look complete different. He was carrying about three times more fat and he had lost most of his muscle mass. He would tell you that just because he stopped training, his muscles did not turn to fat. He knew that this isn't even possible!  He knew that his body stored fat for times of famine and food shortage and when he stopped working out he reduced his muscle mass which was his furnace for burning excess calories.  Fat and muscle are completely independent of each other and the body knows what is fat and what is muscle.  My body building friend's body now required fewer calories so his body began storing the calories as fat.

Remember to maintain a pound of muscle most require an additional 50 calories a day.  There is no way that fat can turn into muscle or vice versa.

## Diet Myth #3

- o Lifting weights and building muscle doesn't help you lose fat.

Again, this is another common myth.  People believe they only need to focus on cardiovascular exercise.  The most important thing to do to avoid weight gain later on is to make sure you have muscle tissue or even to increase your muscle mass.

If you severely cut calories, you will lower your set point and lose muscle tissue; therefore some form of weight bearing exercise is recommended.

To avoid rebound weight, build some muscle. Remember that muscle is very important to keep your metabolism revved like a well oiled engine.

Weight lifting is crucial to keeping your body fit and lean. Another positive result of lifting weights or a good workout routine is that your metabolism is raised for a full 24 hours after you finish.

Many people believe that if women start lifting weights they will look like the women in the body building magazine and they will look too muscular!

Now there are many documented reasons why this is false:

- Women simply do not manufacture the same amount of muscle building hormone testosterone as men. In fact men have 10 times more testosterone than women. If a woman is concerned about her muscles looking bigger, than she can reduce the amount of weight she is lifting and perform more repetitions. In truth, muscle is very dense so if a woman has increased her muscle mass while losing the fat, she will look infinitely smaller and more fit than she did before!

- o Many people believe that most bodybuilders spend all of their time lifting weights, taking steroids and other muscle enhancing drugs. This simply is not true. Some people are just genetically gifted and it doesn't take them as much effort to stay in great shape. However, I do know this many bodybuilders do exercise properly and eat healthy food.

- o To increase muscle mass, it does take a lot of food. Muscle requires a lot of energy and to rebuild damaged muscle (after a workout) eating protein is a must. You see muscle requires a calorie surplus and fat requires a calorie deficit! For this very reason many bodybuilders have two seasons. In the off season, they eat like horses to put as much weight on as possible. Then as the season progresses to contest time, they strip off all of the fat they have put on during the off season by reducing their calorie intake and exercising.

o During the contest season, male bodybuilders and fitness models will reduce their body fat down to 4-6% and the female bodybuilders and fitness models will reduce their body fat down to 8-12%.

o I don't recommend this because this puts a lot of strain on the body. This yo-yo dieting taxes the body and many bodybuilders end up having chronic diseases because they have played havoc on their metabolism.

o However, this does give us the information that if you weight train and do some form of cardio and give the body proper nutrition you will stay lean and fat free...

## Diet Myth #4

### Certain foods, like grapefruit, celery, or broths, can burn fat and make you lose weight.

No foods can burn fat. Some foods with caffeine may increase your metabolism (the way your body utilizes energy or calories) for a short time, but they do not cause a sustained weight loss.

It is still a proven concept that best way to lose weight is to cut back on the intake of calories you eat and become more physically active.

## Diet Myth #5

### Natural or herbal weight loss products are safe and effective.

A weight loss product that makes the claim to be "natural" or "herbal" is not necessarily a safe weight loss product. These products are usually not scientifically tested to prove the marketing assertions they are safe or that they work. For example, herbal products containing ephedra have caused serious health problems and even death. Newer products that claim to be ephedra-free are not necessarily danger-free, because they may contain ingredients similar to ephedra.

Discuss with your health care provider before using any weight loss product. Some natural or herbal weight loss products may actually be harmful.

### *Diet Myth #6*

### *Low-fat or nonfat means no calories.*

Most any low-fat or nonfat food is often lower in calories than the same size portion of the full-fat product.  But <u>many</u> processed low-fat or nonfat foods have just as many calories as the full-fat version of the same food and some even have more calories. They may contain added sugar, flour, or starch thickeners to improve flavor and texture after fat is removed in order to improve the taste. These ingredients add calories.

Understanding the Nutrition Facts Label on a food package to find out how many calories are in a serving is good habit to develop. And always, check the serving size too it may be less than you normally eat.  Some cereals actually get down to counting how many units are in a serving.  Counted your flakes lately?  Just be aware.

## *Diet Myth #7*

### *Skipping meals is a good way to lose weight.*

Studies show that people who skip breakfast and eat fewer times during the day tend to be heavier and have weight management problems than people who eat a healthy breakfast. This may be because people who skip meals tend to feel hungrier later on, and eat more than they normally would. It is because be that eating many small meals throughout the day helps people control their appetites and cravings.

Eating small meals and several snacks throughout the day that include a variety of healthy, low-fat, low-calorie foods is the smart way to take control of your weight loss plan.

## *Diet Myth #8*

### *Eating after 8 p.m. causes weight gain.*

It does not matter what time of day you eat. It is what you eat and how much you eat in addition to how much physical activity you do during the whole day that determines whether you gain, lose, or maintain your weight. No matter when you eat, your body will store extra calories as fat.

If you want to have a snack before bedtime, recount first about how many calories you have consumed that day. And try to avoid snacking in front of the TV at night it may be easier to overindulge when you are mesmerized by the television.

### *Diet Myth #9*

### *Lifting weights is not good to do if you want to lose weight, because it will make you "bulk up."*

Lifting weights or doing strengthening activities like push-ups and any activity on a regular basis can actually help you maintain and lose weight. These activities can help you build muscle, and muscle just burns more calories than body fat.  So if you have more muscle, you burn more calories—even while you're are sitting still. Doing strengthening activities 2 or 3 days a week will not "bulk you up." Only concentrated strength training, combined with a certain genetic background, can build really large muscles.

In addition to doing at least thirty minutes of moderate-intensity physical activity (such as walking two miles in thirty minutes) on most days of the week, try to do strengthening activities two to three days a week. There are several activities that you can do:

- Lift free weights or Nautilus weight machines

- Use resistance bands (large rubber bands )
- Do push-ups or sit-ups
- Do household or garden tasks that make you lift, dig and move
- Walking is the universal activity that always helps
- Biking is the other

# CHAPTER TWELVE

## Dump the Weight For Good This Time!

*You can lose the weight permanently by starting with your mind!*

Through education and sound knowledge, you now know how your body burns fat, stores fat and this means you are in the strong position to finally shed your unwanted weight once and for all.

- ○ Knowing how to recognize fad diets, and how to avoid them means you're so much more ahead of the game than you were before. You'll not be tempted to fall for these fly by night diets that promise "Heaven On Earth" and deliver nothing but disappointment.

You have had years of addictive eating, which got you where you are in the first place, so IT WILL TAKE YOU MORE THAN A WEEK OF DIETING TO CHANGE THIS! IT CAN BE DONE AND YOU CAN DO IT! Remember the Band Aid Solution is temporary solution and it is a lifetime of struggle! So now you finally have the answers you need to really to it this time. Take a deep breath and know you have already come along way baby!

As you know, weight loss is so much more than just the weight itself. Weight Loss is a holistic mindset, because it goes deeper than just the issue of weight in itself. It includes the drives and motivations about how you got here in the first place. Therefore to shed the weight once and for all, it requires some serious introspection and actions. It is not just about physical weight; it is about your mindset!

## *Inches or Pounds?*

Which is more important? If we are on a weight loss program, we become obsessed with the scales. We weigh ourselves everyday or more sometimes and we become discouraged and annoyed when the little hasn't shifted. Suddenly the whole diet success plan is based upon that single measurement. You might weigh yourself before you eat or after you hit the restroom! Please do not let the scale define your weight loss efforts and allow it to make you a basket case!

Yes, weighing yourself is important as a starting point. The most beneficial way is to weigh yourself every two weeks or once a month.
It is too easy to become obsessed with the movement of the needle, or if it's digital you start measuring every tenth of a pound.  Focus on your plan and measure your success by knowing you are meeting your goals at every meal.  The weight will come off and you will be so much more pleased with yourself.

I know, it sounds like torture but it'll prevent you from becoming a slave to the scale! Before you know it you'll be successful with your new Lifestyle Change enough to trust the numbers that the scale shows you.

Do not give your power away to a bit of lifeless machinery.  This is too much power to have over your life!  Your weight will fluctuate throughout the day depending upon what you eat and your fluid intake. Sometimes your body will hold onto more liquid and other days it will delete the liquid.  The body knows how to regulate your fluids in order to maintain a healthy temperature for you, to eliminate toxins and so on. So why on earth would you allow a scale to dictate what your body knows best!

## *The Best Indicator Of Your Weight Is How Your Clothes Fit.*

You may have 5 or more different weight fluctuations throughout the day which makes you feel as if you aren't succeeding with your weight loss.

Your scale can even show you that you have gained weight if you have gained more lean muscle mass. Fat is lighter than muscle. Have you ever noticed that when cleaning out a pan that was filled with fat, the fat floats to the top of the dishwater? This is because fat is lighter than water, so doesn't it stand to reason that you can weigh less but be fatter than someone with lean muscle mass?

Just imagine your horror when the scale shows you have gained 2 lbs. because you don't understand how the body works. Just imagine the elation you feel when you are swimming in your clothes. Doesn't it make sense to trust what your clothes are telling you than the scale?

Remember lean muscle mass weighs more than fat.  In a group research, the results showed that those who adopted a healthy lifestyle change not

only reduced their risk of developing diabetes by 55%, it also showed that the changes in the body where the reflected on the scale.  They had significantly more lean muscle mass and less fat, but the scale didn't show a significant weight loss in pounds.

My advice is this; hide your scale and let your clothes be the indication of how much fat you lose!  Your healthy and toned body will take up much less space and this is what you want!

Why Diets Don't Work

# CHAPTER THIRTEEN

# Self-Improvement Through Self-Motivation

## *Goals And Objectives Are Critical*

I n order to be happy and satisfied, one needs to be motivated. Motivation basically gives us the hope to look ahead and dream higher. It is the force that propels us to go ahead. But why do we need to change? People change for various reasons. Some change because they don't want to face the pain in their lives. Some change because they are sick of their failures. For instance; poor grades can make us realize the importance of hard work while studying and can motivate us to change. Similarly, debts can makes us look for other jobs or manage out finances better

This world is full of negativity and regardless of what people say we need to embrace this negativity and change it. But it is you who has to make this decision! Who is in charge of your life, you or your surroundings? Once, you decide that you are in charge of whatever happens, you will put your foot down and change the things that don't work in your life.

It is easy for people to remain in the shelter of the comfort zone. Have you ever tried stepping out of your comfort zone and taking a sneak peek into what lies beyond? What exactly prevents you from doing so? Fear? Shame? Guilt? Failure?

To improve you must first set your intention (goal) and set some objectives. If you don't know where you are going, you can't get there. Once you know where you are headed, you can easily maintain your focus and not be distracted by anything that hinders your path.

Next, set a concrete plan which will enable you to go for the gold! When planning, know that this could be outside of your comfort zone. However, step out, get into the game. Identify your limitations, your challenges and decide to overcome them. Many have said to think outside of the box but I have also heard it said that you should think inside the box and expand on it. Whatever way you want to look at develop a plan so you can stick to it. You can always change your intention, adjust it and adopt ideas that could take you faster and more efficiently toward it.

Remember you are the owner of your mind. If someone says something to you that you don't like and you become upset. Ask yourself, "Why does this affect me? It is true?" If it isn't just say thank you, I've got it handled!

You can't avoid negative thoughts and people. So change your perception and reframe anything that doesn't carry you toward your goal. We all want approval, control and safety. However, if you seek these wants outside of you, someone can take it away. So, ask yourself if you become upset, "What do I want here, approval, control or safety?" When you define it, stop looking for it outside of yourself; rather give it to yourself by saying,

"I am loved and approved of, I am in control and I am safe." This is an awesome technique to keep you focused on an incredible life which becomes content and happier.

When you are happy and content, your mind works faster and success will come your way. So hold on hard to your dreams, take control of your life and set compass to enjoy the journey with a newer you

Overcoming difficult situations tends to impart a positive feeling that increases your motivation. It may test your patience but it also makes you stretch boundaries. Engaging in healthy situations that test your comfort zone helps to build a stronger psyche.

The empowered mindset is so important. Continuous re-conditioning of your core resonance (your inner self) is paramount to your success. Even if we don't believe we are confident, empowered and whole; if we say it to re-condition our belief system, it becomes a fact. A quote from the Bible in Luke starts out: Act as if . . . .

We are all endowed with a strong character; however we are afraid of our power, so we many times act small as not to offend others. Mahatma Ghandi once said, "Your being small does not serve the world?" Remember this and take the challenge to live up to your full potential!

# CHAPTER FOURTEEN

# The Real Truth About Hypnosis

## *Does it work for Weight Loss?*

In today's world, eating disorders are becoming more commonplace. From anorexia to bulimia to the clinically obese! We are seeing many, many variations of eating disorders.

There is an answer to all of this and it is visualization, mental imaging and hypnosis. We now have enough solid scientific evidence about hypnosis for weight loss to recommend it.

## *Does Hypnosis Really Work for Weight Loss?*

Hypnosis is not a quick fix solution. Hypnosis is used for so many things but it is a gradual re-programming technique for your brain. Just like you won't walk out of a doctor's office and instantly be thinner the same goes for hypnosis.  Hypnosis will allow you to change the faulty programming that has made you choose the wrong foods and adopt unhealthy programs for your weight loss efforts.

Hypnosis re-programs the subconscious mind where you hold your permanent memory, emotions, beliefs and even your creative ideas.  This is what drives your decisions.  Most people think it is the conscious mind that drives you to make decisions when this simply is not true.  We make decisions emotionally and justify logically.  The subconscious mind is considered the emotional mind.

For example:  You have a see a piece of chocolate cake.  You know consciously that it is not in your healthy food group.  However, emotional you think that the chocolate cake will taste good and that would feel good.  So logic (conscious mind decision) flies out the window in the face of emotion (subconscious mind decision).  You choose to eat the cake.

Yes, hypnosis can retrain your brain to make healthy choices and walk away from choices that don't carry you toward your goal.

## *How Effective Is Hypnosis For Weight Loss?*

A Mayo Clinic study by Katherine Zeratsky, RDD, LDD determined that hypnosis can help you shed extra pounds when used with other weight loss methods like diet and exercise. Hypnosis is an altered state of consciousness, usually achieved with the help of a hypnotherapist using verbal rehearsal and mental imagery. When you are under hypnosis, your attention is highly focused and you're more receptive to suggestions, including behavior changes that can help you lose weight. With proper instruction, you can also try self-hypnosis for weight loss. Weight loss hypnosis is usually combined with cognitive behavior therapy.

Through the years, several studies evaluated the use of weight loss hypnosis. Most of the studies found positive, but modest weight-loss results, with an average weight loss of about six pounds. But the quality of some of these studies has been questioned, making it difficult to determine how effective weight loss hypnosis is.

The key to weight loss success is how closely you follow a healthy plan. This is why doctors and nutritionists recommend this Hypnosis Program for Diet Adherence and Lifestyle Change.

Researchers from Tufts-New England Medical Centre (Journal of the American Medical Association, Jan 2005) conducted a study of 4 popular diets.  They determined that the key to successful weight loss isn't the diet itself, but actually _FOLLOWING THE DIET_!

The one-year study of 160 obese adults, who were divided into four diet groups, revealed that the following diets worked marginally.

1.  Weight Watchers (low calorie)
2.  The Zone Diet (low glycemic index)
3.  The Ornish diet (low fat)
4.  Atkins Diet (low carb)

All the diets worked when the participants in the study followed them.  The problem was that in less than one in four could stay on their given diet for the year. It should be noted that the hardest diet to follow was Atkins, followed by the Ornish Diet.  According to the study authors, "no single diet produced satisfactory adherence rates." "

So instead of looking for the "perfect diet," it makes much more sense to find a safe way to adhere to your diet. You'll discover that hypnosis is by far the safest, most researched and effective way for you to stick to any eating plan you have chosen.

Matt Hoover, NBC's The Biggest Loser
Season 2 Winner
on losing weight with hypnosis:

_"I've lost thirty-five pounds already, and I continue to lose an average of 2.3 Three pounds of ugly fat in each week. I finally feel I've control over my desires, thanks to Hypnosis"_

# The Secret Ingredients to Permanent Weight Loss

**Here is the big secret: you have to train your mind to ENJOY sticking to your plan. Whatever healthy plan you choose, it is likely that you are going to have to:**

- **Eat fewer high-sugar or high-fat foods** (reduce your chocolate cake allowance!)

- **Reduce your overall caloric intake**, based on the system you are following

- **Exercise consistently** (whether adding daily walks, or beginning a weight training program)

- **Monitor your progress** in a systematic way

- **Drink more water**, as opposed to sodas and beverages high in sugar

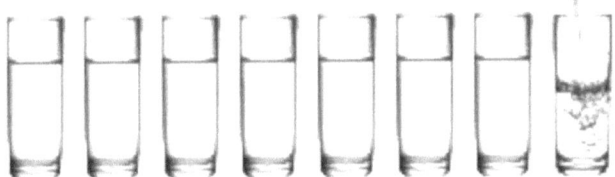

- **Eat more green vegetables**

- **Plan your meals** (and this includes breakfast!)

- **Appreciate yourself and your progress**

Now imagine if there was a proven, well-researched method, **approved by the American Medical Association** that would actually make you WANT to do these things?

Imagine these behaviors **becoming second nature, not an effort.**

# Clinical Hypnosis:

## *The Answer You've Been Looking For!*

## *It's So Easy, It's Like Magic*

Think about a magician - when you see a magician's performance of his or her illusion, it's seamless. You don't "see" how the magic works – it's just works. Reality (just like losing and controlling your weight) is much more complicated.  The magician doesn't just come on stage and perform the illusion. He or she worked hard, doing research, creating or buying the right equipment, developing a performance technique, and then practice, evaluation and repetition.  Yes, rinse and repeat!

Losing and controlling weight appears to be just about willpower — willing something to take place — but really it's about the preparation, the practice, the failure, planning, etc. Weight loss is more about power than willpower. You need to give yourself the power to lose weight.

## Get the Winning Mindset

When you decide to lose weight, you must accept the fact that you must change your lifestyle forever.  Going on and off diets disrupts your metabolism so when you pick up your old habits, you'll find the weight comes back twice as fast.  It destroys your determination and willpower as you keep repeating failure.

So instead of trying to flatten the stomach for Hawaii vacation, or look good for an upcoming wedding, why not set your goals for long term?

## *Power Up Your Mindset*

***If there was one thing I want to stress more than anything else for dieters, is the power of the mind to change the body. Not in a metaphysical "woo-woo" way, but rather in a practical, scientific, measurable way.***

For example, researchers asked a group of basketball players to visualize free throws. They didn't allow them to practice the shots - just think about it, live, in their minds every night. After twelve weeks in a split-group test, where a group of players practiced physical free throws and the other group only mentally practiced, BOTH groups IMPROVED their free throw percentages with very little difference between those who physically shot the ball, and those who just thought of it.

A group of hotel maids were told (wrongly) that their workload met the requirements for weight loss. These women were compared with women who never told this lie. But the women who believed in it, (the group who were told their work would help them lose weight) a significant weight loss was reported, while no weight loss was reported in the other group.

## <u>Hopefully, we have your attention now!</u>
### This is the simple, proven effective, time tested solution, boils down to this:

## Change Your Mind And Your Feelings And Your Behaviors Will Follow!

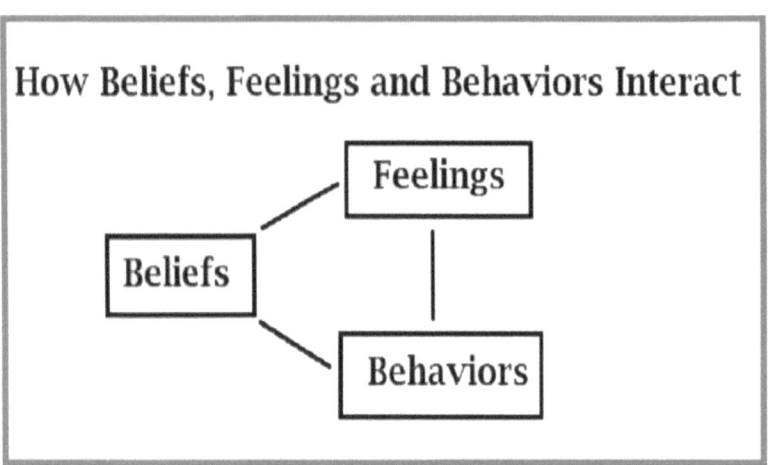

Our lifestyle approach focuses on the mental aspect of weight loss,   combined with the natural healing power of good nutrition and an active body. The Hypnotize Myself Thin program is structured to reduce mental stress and reprogram your inner self to achieve your weight loss goals.

It is a process that has you imagine your dream body, change your neuro-pathways, and create healthy eating habits, so you can reach your ideal weight faster. Why not let us help you "reprogram" your subconscious mind to achieve your weight loss goals and find your fit and trim body in a healthy and natural way?

# You're On Your Way To

# Freedom From Dieting Forever!

# Weight Loss Support

You can find our individual weight, fitness information and solutions available at the following areas:

www.HypnotizeMyselfThin.com
www.FreedomFromDietingForever.com
www.facebook.com/HypnotizeMyselfThin
and Checkout my Success Seminars
http://www.codyhortonsuccessseminars.com/

We hope you found our book enjoyable and informative and hope you reach out through our websites and let us know what you think.

Check out our new Affirmations For Weight Loss
And the new series of solutions offered by affirmations.

Best Wishes,
**Cody Horton, Ph.D.**
  **Clinical Hypnotherapist, Certified Homeopath**

**Daniel E. Vance B.S.**
  **Physical Fitness, Nutritional Wellness.**

www.ingramcontent.com/pod-product-compliance
Lightning Source LLC
Chambersburg PA
CBHW020243290526
45784CB00003B/1088